BUSTED!

An Uplifting Breastimony of god's grace

BY KAREN BAREFOOT

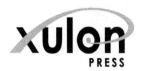

CSSS~

Dedicated to the Great Physician
and the wonderful earthly physicians
He provided for me, as well as my
amazing husband, Don, who nursed me
back to health in a multitude of ways.

"You restored me to health and let me live."
Isaiah 38:16

Putting the "CAN" in Cancer

When Jesus asks you,

"Can you trust me when I say that in all things I work for the good of those who love Me?"

You can say, "Yes, I <u>can, Sir</u>."

"Do you believe that I will heal you in My way and in My time?"

You can say, "Yes, I <u>can, Sir</u>."

"Can you rest in Me, receive My peace, and still have joy in your present circumstances?"

You can say, "Yes, I <u>can, Sir</u>."

"Lord, thank You for carrying me through this and giving me strength to persevere."

"God is our refuge and strength, an ever-present help in trouble. Therefore we will not fear... The LORD Almighty is with us."
Psalm 42:1,2,11

Contents

INTRODUCTION

❦

Most everyone gets that sinking feeling simply *hearing* the word "Cancer". Some can't even say the word, but just call it "the big C". For *me*, "the big C" turned into "the Big See". Throughout my cancer journey I could *See* God in very **BIG** ways! He revealed areas where He had already gone before me and laid the stepping stones that I would need to step on to follow Him along this unblazed trail I had just found myself on. He showed up every step of the way with sign posts that gave me direction, lookout points for me to stop and see His beauty, and places to rest peacefully in His love. With my faith in Jesus Christ as my compass and the Bible as my map, we walked together along this winding path until we reached the summit where I could yell out, *"I'm free! Cancer Free!"*

I hope my use of God's Word out of context doesn't offend anyone. I have the highest regard for Scripture, but there *are* some funny phrases within the pages of His Word. I truly believe it when He says:

> *"As the rain and the snow*
> *come down from heaven,*
> *and do not return to it*
> *without watering the earth*

---

and making it bud and flourish,
so that it yields seed for the sower
and bread for the eater,
so is my word that goes out from
my mouth: It will not return to me empty,
but will accomplish what I desire and achieve
the purpose for which I sent it."
Isaiah 55:10-11

So He can even use my occasional humorous usage of His Word for His glory.

I hope you'll grab your walking stick and join me on my journey through "the Big See".

"Come and see what the LORD has done,
His awesome deeds for mankind!" Psalm 66:5

~ 1 ~

C CHANGE

One of the current buzz words in the business world lately is Sea Change. It means "a gradual transformation in which the form is retained but the substance is replaced", or, "substantive or significant change". My life has been a gradual transformation by many significant **C** Changes.

I can divide my life into three distinct divisions: **C**hildren, **C**hrist, and this newest **C** Change. These three events in my life were gigantic forks in the road for me where my life was irrevocably changed forever.

Anyone who has been blessed with **C**hildren knows what a dramatic change it is in every area of your life. There is no more "me". Everything becomes "we".

When our son, Brandon, was a senior in high school and ready to head off to college, **C**hrist came into my life and I fell head-over-heels in love with Him. Soon, God replaced my empty nest with "my cup runneth over".

While those first two events brought joy and new purpose to my life, this third "**C**" came in like a tsunami, bringing with it wave after wave of death and destruction to my soul. It was as if a bomb had gone off in my life and I was wandering around shell-shocked.

Up until this **C** Change, my life was as close to perfect as you could get. Well, alright, I'll admit; we did own two demon-possessed wire-haired fox terrorists as pets and I was crazy enough to get braces on my teeth for two years at the age of 50, but that's about it.

Then November 2007 hit and the walls came tumblin' down. For almost 2½ years solid, one thing after another, *all starting with the letter C*, crashed in on me. I was "C sick"! And all of this happened during the most severe case of *mental*pause a woman can go through! Just ask my husband, Don! I'm sure he wondered many nights coming home from work whether a helmet and flak jacket would be more appropriate attire than his flimsy three piece suit! It's a good thing we didn't own a gun, because I definitely would've threatened him with it if he even walked close to the thermostat! I used to say, "Sometimes I need to take a nap just to get away from myself!" God is not fair. He's good, sovereign, almighty, and loving toward all He's made, but He is **not** fair...at least not from our self-centered human per-spective. I spent 43 years of my life in the Midwest freezing my tail off nine months of the year, then we moved to warm North Carolina just in time to start menopause. Who would have thought I'd miss snow storms in May or seeing my breath on a September morning?!

There were at least eight major "C"s that hit around the same time. I won't go into all of them, but one of the big "C"s was cancer. No, not mine, that would come later.

Our only child, Brandon (age 30 at the time), called us in early December of 2007 and said, "I was mowing the lawn today and had a terrible stomach pain, so I laid down for a while. But Jenn's (Brandon's wife) mom said I had better go to the emergency room just in case it's my appendix. So I went and they did a scan and found a baseball-size mass on my stomach." It turned out to be a malignant sarcoma. Although they account for only 1% of all cancers, sarcomas are some of the scariest and hardest to treat cancers out there. He had surgery, followed by "Draino®-strength" chemotherapy and is now a healthy, happy dad of three-year-old twin boys! What a testimony of their trust in God; even though the prognosis for his cancer was questionable at best, Brandon and Jenn went forward in faith and decided to start their family. The twins were conceived from the frozen sperm he banked before his chemo and were born quite prematurely. What a bunch of fighters! Brandon and his two sons are literally my three miracles (and Jenn's strength through all of their trials is a miracle, too!) and have brought sunshine to my life in a way that is indescribable!!! If you aren't a grandparent yet, you are missing God's reward for surviving parenthood!

Even though Brandon's cancer was a trial that no parent *ever* wants to watch their child endure, I had a peace from God that he would be healed. It was the relational fallout from several of the other "**C**"s during that period of time that took its toll on me and simply had a strangle-hold on my heart and mind. Satan had dug a pit and I fell into it and couldn't get out. I vividly remember one day sitting there having one of my many pity parties, saying to myself, "It will be a miracle if I don't get some kind of illness. You just can't be stressed and depressed for this long before your body rebels."

I prayed and pleaded with God to rescue me, but He was working something in me that couldn't be acquired by having a "perfect" life. I was in the Refiner's fire and He was watching me closely so I would not be burned up while

He carefully skimmed the impurities off the top of my life. Eventually I will become pure gold (the day I enter heaven!), but I can promise you, it's hotter than you-know-where while you're in the midst of it. But, I was used to the heat. My hot flashes could rival a fiery furnace any day!!!

> *"In this you greatly rejoice, though now for a little while you may have had to suffer grief in all kinds of trials. These have come so that your faith ~ of greater worth than gold, which perishes, even though refined by fire ~ may be proved genuine and may result in praise, glory and honor when Jesus Christ is revealed."* 1 Peter 1:6-7

So, during this time, all I could do was climb up into my Heavenly Father's lap and snuggle close to His heart...right where He wanted me. Yes, thankfully there was one "**C**" that lit my way out of the darkness: **C**hrist!

I tend to wander off on my own, full speed ahead, so sure that I'm on the highway to happiness. But, in all three "**C** changes" of my life, God brought me to a place where He **proved** that it was not ME running the show, but Him. I was too hard-headed to notice Him when we were raising Brandon. But, when the Nerf bat doesn't work, God uses something a little heftier —like a two-by-four— to drive you to your knees! In all three cases, He stripped me of everything I thought was making me happy, as well as, things that I was so sure of. He **will not** share His throne with anyone, but that doesn't stop us from trying to wiggle our way onto it, hoping He won't mind sharing it with us occasionally. But He *does* mind.

I love word pictures. There is a particularly brutal picture that is precious to me. In ancient days, if a sheep tended to wander off frequently, the shepherd would break one of its legs, causing it to be helpless on its own. Then he would carry that sheep on his shoulders, making the sheep totally dependent on the shepherd for every need. Once the leg healed, the sheep knew the safest place is near the shepherd and didn't wander away again.

That was me! Before I met Christ, I was so happy doing life on my terms, not knowing my "perfect" life was missing the one thing that really mattered: Jesus! As any parent knows, sometimes you have to hold your child's face in your hands for them to look directly at you and focus on what you're saying. God sometimes needs to do that with us to get our attention. We have to remember that if we're followers of Jesus, God doesn't punish us, He disciplines us. There is a big difference. Hebrews 12:7-11 says:

"Endure hardship as discipline; God is treating you as sons. For what son is not disciplined by his father? If you are not disciplined (and everyone undergoes discipline), then you are illegitimate children and not true sons. Moreover, we have all had human fathers who disciplined us and we respected them for it. How much more should we submit to the Father of our spirits and live! Our fathers disciplined us for a little while as they thought best; but God disciplines us for our good, that we may share in his holiness. Later on, however, it produces a harvest of righteousness and peace for those who have been trained by it."

As God's Word says, *"No discipline seems pleasant at the time, but painful."* Nobody asks for trials, but most everybody says that that's where they felt closest to the Lord and learned so many lessons through their particular refining process.

15

I'll wrap up this chapter by sharing my turning point in this latest **C** Change. This will sound strange to most. Believe me; it was *really* strange to me, too. I am not one who claims to hear from God audibly, but this episode was as real as if He had been sitting right next to me. It's never happened before this, or since, but it was life-changing for me. This **C** is Clay.

Don and I were driving to another state one evening and it was like a movie started playing in my head that *I* didn't initiate. I couldn't stop it or alter it. I tried, but it just kept going. It was the story of the Potter's House in Jeremiah 18:1-4. I had never studied that passage per se, but I knew there were several passages in the Bible where God is portrayed as the Potter and we are the clay. The passage reads:

> *"This is the word that came to Jeremiah from the LORD: "Go down to the potter's house, and there I will give you my message." So I went down to the potter's house, and I saw him working at the wheel. But the pot he was shaping from the clay was marred in his hands; so the potter formed it into another pot, shaping it as seemed best to him."*

God spoke to my heart, "You are so focused on the smashed blob of clay, that you aren't seeing that I am making you into a new pot that is more like what *I* want you to be." That rattled me to my core, but it changed my entire outlook from that point on. Sometimes God has to smash us so He can transform us into a better 'pot' than the old one.

Instead of the *illusion* of a "perfect" pot that was the old me, I now have cracks and holes in my new pot. God designed my new pot to be that way; it wasn't an accident. In Matthew 5:14-16, Jesus (who calls Himself "The Light of the World") tells His followers,

"You are the light of the world. A city on a hill cannot be hidden. Neither do people light a lamp and put it under a bowl. Instead they put it on its stand, and it gives light to everyone in the house. In the same way, let your light shine before men, that they may see your good deeds and praise your Father in heaven."

Those cracks and holes in our clay pots are there to shine *CHRIST's* light to others and that we will all give our praises to God the Father. That glory belongs to Him, not us. Sometimes we need to be reminded of that. I know I do. So, I'm getting used to my new "earthen vessel", but I sure don't have everything down pat by any stretch of the imagination. At times I still try to cover up my cracks and holes so I don't look so imperfect, but then I am reminded that Christ's light can't shine through me when I do that. So now I simply take it as a compliment when I'm accused of being a crackpot and just keep on shining!

"Shine like stars in the universe as you hold out the word of life." Philippians 2:15-16

~2~

THE BEND IN THE ROAD

❦

S o, were you wondering, "I thought this book was about her breast cancer journey"? Well, the bridge from there to here began in January, 2011 when I told Don that the black cloud of depression had finally lifted and I felt like me again (The Potter & the Clay 'movie' had happened about six months prior to this). That oppressive feeling had lifted and I felt so free. I was ready to tackle the world with *real* joy again.

So many good things happened that spring, including finally selling our house after having it on the market for almost six years (That alone would make most people depressed!). Three days after moving I spent four weeks helping my parents move into a retirement community. It was hard work, but we had a ball! We were also able to spend time with our grandbabies, or, as my friend calls them, our "baby grands".

My journey reminds me of one of the funniest/most embarrassing stories we tell about when we lived in Chicago. One night we went out to dinner with friends and they were following us to the restaurant. Don is a really fast and "sporting" driver. He looked in the rearview mirror to see if the couple was still behind us. At that very moment, the road took a 90 degree turn and we didn't!! We went airborne and bounced over a bunch of railroad tracks in an old rail yard. We just sat there stunned for a few seconds, backed the car over the tracks again, got back on the road and went on our way again.

That was similar to how we felt about my cancer diagnosis. My health has been great all these years, then, out of the blue came this sharp bend in the road!

In December of 2010 I had a routine mammogram and the doctor saw a tiny line (I mean *really* tiny) that looked like a little grain of rice. She wanted to look at it again in six months, so at the end of June they did another mammogram. I never once thought about it in the interim. I haven't had any serious health issues as an adult and I don't even take any medications, so I was in total agreement with the doctor when she said, "I'm sure it's nothing, but I'd like to do a biopsy just to make sure." Later that week I went in for this "routine, minimally invasive procedure".

My first "God moment" in all this was when I showed up for my appointment and the receptionist said, "Would you like to pay the full $1600 today?" The shock on my face must have freaked her out... or maybe I should say, the freaked out look on *my* face shocked *her*. She said, "Didn't they tell you that? Someone was supposed to have gone over all this with you already." I KNOW God hid that from me until it was too late to turn back because I would have *never* spent that kind of money out of my own pocket given that that tiny little line on the mammogram was "nothing".

The phrase "Ignorance is Bliss" was certainly true in the case of this routine biopsy. No wonder they don't warn you about this kind of stuff beforehand... so ladies, you have been forewarned. When they say, "you'll feel some pressure", think 'being shot at point blank range by a meat thermometer'! Holy Cow! (I actually said that when she skewered me!)

Thus began my cancer journey.

WARNING!! Before you read another word of this, I have to give you a heads-up on what to expect. When the word gets out that you have breast cancer, people come out of the woodwork with their stories. Some truly are there to help answer your concerns, but many of them *have* to tell you the horror story of their friend or relative that had cancer. Some people will tell you to call a friend of theirs that has gone through "the same *exact* breast cancer you have". Even though they are only trying to help, you need to be careful. I found that after talking to a few women who supposedly had "exactly the same kind of cancer that you have", they weren't the same at all. I received such a lesson in Cancer 101 going through this; very few cancer patients are "just like you". I talked to women who had much more invasive, higher stage cancer than me that didn't have to do any adjuvant therapy (that's the fancy name for any follow-up treatments such as chemotherapy or radiation). Why did I have "the best kind of breast cancer" at only a Stage 0 (ending up at a Stage 1A after the final pathology reports came back) and have to have chemo, Herceptin and an anti-estrogen pill for 5 years?! So, my suggestion is, only talk to a select few people who will answer *your* questions. There are dozens of different factors that the doctors have to take into account to give **you** the right diagnosis and treatment.

From here on out, I will tell *my* tale through my email/ CaringBridge® updates. Below are the two emails I sent out to friends and family that first week:

Hmmmm (7/17/11)

...I have to focus on a new "adventure". I had a mammogram and they found a tiny white line, so they did a biopsy and it is a calcification that is pre-cancerous, but probably would turn into cancer later if nothing was done with it. It's called Ductal Carcinoma In Situ (DCIS). They said if you have to get breast cancer, this is the one you want. It is only two mm long (about the size of a grain of rice), and they removed a bunch of it in the biopsy. Long story short, they are talking about doing a lumpectomy and 5 days of radiation twice a day. I have my first appointment for an MRI tomorrow, then see the oncologist on Tuesday. I'll keep you posted as I learn more. I am not worried in the least... I have a God who has this all planned out, so I just have to keep my eyes on Him for direction and a bit of hand-holding. Obviously, I desire your prayers, but no worrying allowed!!!

WHAT?! (7/19/11)

Well, I found out why nobody calls me Doctor Barefoot... because I stink at diagnosing medical issues! That "I'm sure it's nothing", turned out to be a much bigger something.

That little "grain of rice" calcification they found in my breast turned out to be a whole bowl of Rice Krispies! The mammogram only showed that one tiny spot, but the MRI yesterday showed that the entire duct is peppered with these calcifications. The doctors have their weekly meeting to discuss all their patients tomorrow morning, so I will be "on the docket", then he will call me to tell me what they want to do. BUT, he told us today that the probable course of action is a mastectomy, not just a lumpectomy. WHAT!?!?!?

So, it looks like I'm going to be busy for the next few months. Yuck.

As I said before, no worrying allowed, but keep me in your prayers. When you see a little ant hill or a fried egg, send up a prayer for me.

As you can guess, I'm not the most well-endowed woman around. Most middle schoolers would laugh at me. I always joked that I'd never get breast cancer because the cancer cells couldn't find them! But, there I was, with breast cancer.

I will tell you up front, I am not a worrier by nature. But, more importantly, I have an unshakeable faith in God, who is sovereign over everything. Even the news of cancer, then the thought of having a mastectomy didn't rattle me. I realize I am not in the majority on this one! Since I became a follower of Jesus (at age 39), I have seen God's faithfulness, His provision for every tiny detail of my life, and that *"His goodness and mercy will follow me all the days of my life."* (Psalm 23:6) He has never left me hanging out there all by myself. Even in those dark three years, He called me to follow Him even closer and let me know He was there every step of the way.

> *"Seek first His kingdom and His righteousness, and all these things will be given to you as well. Therefore do not worry about tomorrow, for tomorrow will worry about itself. Each day has enough trouble of its own."* Matthew 6:33-34

Many Bible teachers say "you can't hold onto faith and fear at the same time." They cannot co-exist. I choose faith because it is there that you see God work out things in ways that only He can do! Those of you who are gripped with fear, you will never experience all that God has for you to learn in that Refiner's fire that I talked about earlier. When you choose fear, you are trying to control the situation on your own. You are trusting in your *self*-sufficiency. You might get through the trial by gritting your teeth all the way through, but you end up only telling a good story in the end. Those who choose faith rely on God to guide us through the storms of life, He shows us what He wants us to learn, and as a result, we can reflect His character and faithfulness to those who don't know Him. We find that God is sufficient and when He has walked us through our trial, we end up telling a **God** story.

"But He said to me, 'My grace if sufficient for you, for My power is made perfect in weakness.' Therefore I will boast all the more gladly about my weaknesses, so that Christ's power may rest on me. That is why, for Christ's sake, I delight in weaknesses, in insults, in hardships, in persecutions, in difficulties. For when I am weak, then I am strong." 2 Corinthians 12:9-10.

I'm not so sure many of us could say that we 'delight' in those things, but if we can learn to accept them, even embrace them because they have been filtered through the hand of God for us, He will be able to use our cancer journey for many purposes.

With my surgery at hand, I wrote to my prayer partners:

Keeping You Abreast (8/5/11)

A friend of mine sent this to me and it is a Scripture passage to hang your hat on!

"They will have no fear of bad news; their hearts are steadfast, trusting in the LORD. Their hearts are secure, they will have no fear; in the end they will look in triumph on their foes." Psalm 112:7-8

Jesus Christ will always be my BFF... *breast* friend forever!

Well, someone in this country has to get some skin in the game and make painful cuts, so I'm going forward with my very own "Cut, Cap and Balance" on August 17th. We met with the cancer surgeon as well as the plastic surgeon this week and they are coordinating the procedure as you are reading this.

In my family we have joked about my Grandma who couldn't be bothered with such nuisances as breast cancer, followed by colon cancer the following year. She just told them "Get it out! I have too much to do." She attributes her health and well-being to being a 'hearty Swede'. Well, just call me Lilli Jr. I told the doctor yesterday that I was available if he wanted to do it during his lunch hour.

I just love how God has given me confirmation at key points along the way. The day I was walking in to my first consultation with Dr. W (surgeon), a woman I had only met twice briefly was coming out of his office. She told me she only had rave reviews for him and that I would love him. Then, yesterday morning while we were at the meeting to talk about all the whens and hows, I received an email from a member of our church who is an anesthesiologist at the hospital where I will have surgery. He also confirmed how "excellent" both of my doctors are. Maybe I'll get him as my anesthesiologist and have the trifecta of excellence!!!

I still have "the peace that passes understanding" that Jesus promised. That's not to say that I'm not a little freaked out about losing a part of me (a very small part, but nonetheless). I can promise you I won't ever pray for God to help me lose weight ever again!

Well, who would've ever guessed that I would be getting breast reduction surgery!?! Or, more specifically, breast de-"duct"-tion.

Truly, I am grateful that God has spared me from a much more severe form of cancer like many who are reading this. I do not take this lightly, but humor is just my way of lightening the situation.

I cherish all your prayers, calls, cards and notes. I am blessed beyond measure knowing that I have friends and family as precious as all of you!

"We who have fled to take hold of the hope offered to us may be greatly encouraged. We have this hope as an anchor for the soul, firm and secure." Hebrews 6:18-19

THE PINK BRA TEAM IS BORN

Pink Bra Team (8/9/11)

I've decided to call you all my "Pink Bra Team" because you are so supportive and you lift me up with your prayers. Not to mention that my cup runneth over with joy that I have so many great people who care for me!!!!

I just had another answer to prayer. Dr. Singer said that he has requested to be my anesthesiologist.

"Let the saints rejoice... and sing for joy on their beds." Psalm 149:5

Several of you have asked about my surgery schedule. It is as follows:

* Arrive groggy as heck at the Surgery Center at 6:45am

* I am scheduled to dye by injection at 8am. (injection of the dye to find my sentinel nodes for the upcoming biopsy during surgery)

* My de-'duct"-tion begins at 8:30

* Around 9:30-10:00, the rebuilding of the temple begins.

* Noon to who-knows-when; say a whole bunch of totally crazy things under the influence of the narcotics and remain even groggier than when I arrived.

* Thank God over and over for His unfailing love and presence in my life!!!

If you're wondering what specific prayers to pray for me, the biggie is that when they do the biopsies on the lymph nodes (during surgery), that they would be perfectly clear. That way I definitely won't have to do any radiation.

> *"Because of the LORD's great love we are not consumed, for His compassions never fail. They are new every morning; great is Your faithfulness. I say to myself, 'The LORD is my portion; therefore I will wait for Him.' The LORD is good to those whose hope is in Him, to the one who seeks Him; it is good to wait quietly for the salvation of the LORD."* Lamentations 3:22-26

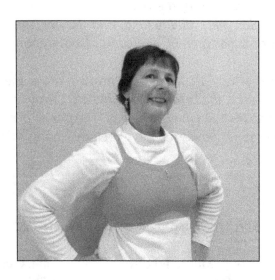

Hospital or Bust! (8/16/11)

Given the choice, I'll keep the bust! But the choice was made for me, so off we go to the Surgical Center in the morning.

"...your end has come, the time for you to be cut off."
Jeremiah 51:13

Don't try visiting me at the hospital because, given my past track record with anesthesia, I will be starring in the reenactment of Rip Van Winkle for days!!!!!

"When you lie down, you will not be afraid; when you lie down, your sleep will be sweet." Proverbs 3:24

I will stay overnight, but will HAVE TO go home the following morning by 8am!! These people obviously don't know or care about my normal sleep schedule! How inconsiderate.

"Let the beloved of the LORD rest secure in Him, for He shields [her] all day long, and the one the LORD loves rests between His shoulders." Deuteronomy 33:1

"And the prayers offered in faith will make the sick person well; the Lord will raise him up... Pray for each other so that you may be healed. The prayer of a righteous man is powerful and effective." James 4:15-16

If you don't have a prayer team, GET ONE NOW!!

We are not meant to go through trials alone. Call out the troops to pray for you. Send out an APB (All Points Bulletin) to everyone you know, and everyone they know, to get them praying for you. Storm the gates of heaven with your petitions! God loves it when He hears your name. Remember, He has your name written on the palm of His hand as a reminder of how special you are! *"See, I have engraved you on the palms of My hands."* Isaiah 49:16. But even if you only have a small "A cup" Pink Bra Team, you have the most powerful prayer partners in the universe, Jesus Himself and the Holy Spirit.

"In the same way, the Spirit helps us in our weakness. We do not know what we ought to pray for, but the Spirit Himself intercedes for us through wordless groans. And He who searches our hearts knows the mind of the Spirit, because the Spirit intercedes for God's people in accordance with the will of God. Christ Jesus...is at the right hand of God and is also interceding for us." Romans 8:26-27, 34

"Therefore He is able to save completely those who come to God through Him because He always lives to intercede for them." Hebrews 7:25

There is an interesting story in the book of Exodus related to having a support system during this time of battling cancer (or any difficult circumstance).

"Moses, Aaron and Hur went to the top of the hill. ***As long as Moses held up his hands, the Israelites were winning, but whenever he lowered his hands, the Amalekites were winning. When Moses' hands grew tired, they took a stone and put it under him and he sat on it. Aaron and Hur held his hands up— one on one side, one on the other—so that his hands remained steady till sunset."*** Exodus 17:10-12

Moses couldn't defeat the enemy by himself, so his close friends came alongside, ministering to him so he would be assured of victory. Notice that when Moses' hands grew tired, they provided comfort and rest for him. Then they held his hands up to steady him until the whole battle was over. They were strong *for* him when he was weak.

The apostle Paul thanked those who assisted him in his work in every letter he wrote. We are no stronger or more capable than Moses or Paul, so why would we think we can go through something as challenging as cancer all by ourselves?! Trust me; I need to preach that to myself! I didn't want to put anybody out. You might be able to relate; "Everybody is so busy and I don't want to impose on anyone." But, that is part of God's plan. He made us to enter into the lives of others, to intertwine our lives, to minister to one another. So when friends offer you help, *allow* them to come and lift up your arms! Let others share in the experience of seeing God give you victory!

"It is God who arms me with strength and makes my way perfect... You give me Your shield of victory, and Your right hand sustains me; You stoop down to make me great." Psalm 18:32,35

~4~

SURPRISE...AGAIN...AND AGAIN!

cover

...And the bREaST is History (8/20/11)

Literally, but we'll be working on that!

"He has sent Me to bind up the brokenhearted (that's right near the breast!)...to bestow on them a crown of beauty instead of ashes, the oil of gladness instead of mourning, and a garment of praise instead of a spirit of despair. They will be called oaks of righteousness, a planting of the LORD for the display of His splendor... All who see them will acknowledge that they are a people the LORD has blessed." Isaiah 61:1,3,9

Oh, how blessed we are indeed!

I received the answer to our prayers last evening. No lymph node involvement, so no radiation, but there was a little surprise. When they did the pathology from the mastectomy, there was a tiny spot that had started to invade the tissue outside of the duct... which no longer makes it a Stage 0 cancer. But the surgeon thought it was so tiny and since we did the mastectomy, he doesn't think that the oncologist will even recommend any chemo. Dr. W (surgeon) is making an appointment so we can discuss the options with the oncologist. But, Dr. W said not to lose focus on the important part, that it is *not* in the lymph nodes. So we will sing praises for our specific answer to that prayer request!

So, looks like more prayers are necessary! Now we'll ask God to have eradicated all of the cancer so I don't have to do any chemo.

I can still continue on with my reconstruction project. I may have to get a pink hardhat! (Don would say I'm hard-headed enough to withstand anything that gets thrown at me! Sometimes that's a good thing!) Once I am healed up, we can start working toward a Cuter Hooter. The plastic surgeon said the whole process will take up to a year to accomplish the desired results.

My recuperation is coming along great! I feel a bit better with each nap, and I'm getting a ton of those! Lots of doctors' appointments next week, but it all gets me closer to feeling "whole" again.

Thank you to all who have loved on us so well. Jesus has been present every day as each of you has been His hands, feet and heart!

I Feel Drained! (9/6/11)

Yea! My drainage tube came out today! That precious little accessory dangling down like the White Rabbit's giant pocket watch was not the best look on me. Not to mention, red is not my color.

*"Let us **throw off everything that hinders** and the sin that so easily entangles, and let us run with*

perseverance the race marked out for us. Let us fix our eyes on Jesus..." Hebrews 12:1-2

My doctor is thrilled with how well I'm doing. I feel so blessed to have such a sweet, caring doctor. We are bosom buddies now.

"I saw the Lord always before me... therefore my heart is glad and my tongue rejoices... You have made known to me the paths of life; You will fill me with joy in Your presence." Acts 2:25-28

The foundation of the temple was laid during the "big" surgery and next Tuesday she begins the rebuilding of the walls. Dr. S said I'm ahead of schedule, which is a kinder, gentler way of saying "since you're only building a tiny temple, it won't take that long to finish." Hey, I'm okay with that. I don't need a mansion... I'm promised that when I get to heaven.

"The day for building your walls will come, the day for extending your boundaries." Micah 7:11

...And Now You Know The bREaST of the Story (9/12/11)

What a wonderful day yesterday was; I went to the medical oncologist and she told me that I don't need to do any radiation, chemo...or anything else. But, it took her an hour and a half to get to that part of the discussion. It was agonizing. The longer she talked, the more nervous I became about what she was going to recommend. I wish she had told us upfront what she had in mind, *THEN* gone through all the detailed analysis. We were mentally exhausted afterwards.

Today Dr. S decided to wait for two weeks to start blowing up the balloon, so the party will have to be put on hold.

"May the God of hope fill you with all joy and peace as you trust in Him, so that you may overflow with hope by the power of the Holy Spirit." Romans 15:13

Okay, somewhere in the fog of information overload at the beginning of all this, I missed a big definition. Dr. S said she was going to use AlloDerm® in the operating room reconstruction project. It sounds like such a nice name, but I just found out that it is cadaver something!! EWWWWWWW!!!! Talk about **DEAD MAM**mary **WALKING!!!**

"The God who gives life to the dead and calls things that are not as though they were." Romans 4:17

My Bubble Has Burst (9/13/11)

No, not that one!

We need to do another lift... a faith lift. More prayer! Yesterday late afternoon the oncologist called and said, "I've been bothered by something in your chart, so I poured over it again. I called the pathologist and we went through your findings." Very long, technical story short, she basically said I think we need to throw the kitchen sink at it. Whaaaaaaat? How did we go from "definitely no chemo, that would be way over the top" to "we need to do 9 weeks of chemo, another IV drug along with it for six months, plus five years of an anti-estrogen drug."? Don't you think she might have done her homework *before* we arrived?

Needless to say, we are getting a second opinion. We can't for the life of us understand why you would do all that for something that was totally removed with clear margins and on and on. I think it's called "covering your butt". I am willing to do whatever treatment is truly necessary, but I'm not crazy about subjecting my body and mind to the "let's kill the ant with a nuclear bomb" method.

"In this you greatly rejoice, though now for a little while you may have had to suffer grief in all kinds of trials. These have come so that your faith — of greater worth than gold, which perishes, even though refined by fire — may be proved genuine and may result in praise, glory and honor when Jesus Christ is revealed." 1 Peter 1:6-7

Dazed and Confused…Still (9/19/11)

We went to the oncologist (Dr. K) again today to hear her out in person. We came out just as confused as before. I'm just going to have to wait for the other opinions before we even think about it again.

"How long will you waver between two opinions?" 1 Kings 18:21

I told Dr. W that I didn't want to work with her, so he said he had worked with an oncologist in Winston-Salem that his patients really liked. He is going to call her office and ask if she would see me. At the least, I'll have a second opinion, then, if I like her I can switch.

As I was driving to get my haircut yesterday, the new oncologist's nurse called saying, "If you can get here ASAP, Dr. H will see you." U-turn! Needless to say, no haircut. She fit me into her schedule on the spur of the moment and Dr. H told me more in 40 minutes than Dr. K did in three visits! I have my peace back knowing I'll be in her care (God's care, through her!). I love this new doctor! She really gave me full

35

confidence just meeting with her yesterday. What an amazing work of God. Thanks for another wonderful gift Lord!!!!!

"I am still confident of this: I will see the goodness of the LORD in the land of the living. Wait for the LORD; be strong and take heart and wait for the LORD." Psalm 27:13-14

Oh, I forgot to mention one of the big reasons I love Dr. H so much. She keeps calling me 'young lady' and every time she talks about this whole process, she says "and because you're still so young..." I mean, seriously, what's a little chemo when you can hear 'sweet nothings' like that every time you go in!!!

"How sweet are your words to my taste, sweeter than honey to my mouth!" Psalm 119:103

Little House of Horrors (9/22/11)

BOOb!

Halloween has come early! How did I go from girl to ghoul in four months? How did I go from "Oh, if you're going to get cancer this is the best kind to have" to this spooky "Wow! This thing is angry, aggressive and scary"? No, *not me*, the cancer!!! How did I go from "Once the cancer is removed, the cancer will be gone for good" to "We need to do chemo, Herceptin, and anti-hormone treatment because this tiny invasion is really nasty"? Obviously God has a different path for me to take.

"In his heart a man plans his course, but the LORD determines his steps." Proverbs 16:9

A friend of mine wrote back from my last email and said, "Maybe God *made* the first oncologist look closer at your pathology report after you left so that she could save your life." I *do* have a God that could easily do that. So, I will look on the bright side of that devastating flip-flop. Maybe *I* will have to do a flip-flop of my own and have her go from Zero to Hero instead of the reverse. I am still monstrously unhappy about it though.

"Though I walk in the midst of trouble, You preserve my life. You stretch out Your hand against the anger of my foes (cancer); with Your right hand You save me." Psalm 138:6-8

The Bible says that our bodies are the temple of the Holy Spirit, but it looks like mine is going to be a haunted house for at least the next six months! Booooooo!

Man, and I was looking so forward to dressing up like the maid with the perky cleavage this Halloween, but it looks more like I will have to settle for the Grim Reaper! Or, the hairless horseman... with chemo brain a strong possibility, I may be the headless horseman after all. Hey, I know, I'll go as a stereotypical blonde; big hooters & no brain...just without the hair.

Darn! It was so much more fun just *talking* about getting cuter hooters!

"But this happened that we might not rely on ourselves but on God, who raises the dead...On Him we have set our hope that He will continue to deliver us, as you help us by your prayers. Then many will give thanks on our behalf for the gracious favor granted us in answer to the prayers of many." 2 Corinthians 1:10-11

There will be many ups and downs in this roller coaster ride. Keep an open mind and heart. As you can see from my story, what I thought was going to happen and what actually did happen were two different things. Don't carve in stone what the doctors say they "think" will happen; that's just their best guess at the time. Every step of the way what I thought was going to happen, or what the doctor thought, changed with new information. Starting with my diagnosis from the mammogram (going from "I'm sure it's nothing to it's something and it's cancer"), to needing a mastectomy instead of a lumpectomy, from "it's all enclosed within the duct, so when we take the tissue out, you will be cancer-free" to the final pathology report showing a very tiny, but nasty invasion just outside the duct, from one day not needing any further treatment to the next day throwing the kitchen sink at it, to putting my breast reconstruction on hold because I *did* have to have chemo, to wondering if my white blood cell count was high enough to get my next treatment. All of these things could have been devastating and depressing if I hadn't had open hands and trusted God with the outcome. Clenched fists around *your* idea of what *should* happen only leads to disappointment and bitterness. And, negative feelings compromise your immune system, leading to all sorts of problems at a time when you are in the greatest need of the vital "fuel" you need to fight this disease. So, keep soaking in the Scriptures to stay positive. There is nothing like reading the promises of God over and over! They will become "good medicine".

~5~

Breast, Test, Blessed

The Phoenix Rises From the Ashes (9/27/11)

Today I expanded my horizons! I was infused with my first saline injection in my expander. I'm no music major, but I can sure tell the difference between an *A flat* and a *B sharp*!! Woo Hoo! I just can't get the old song by the Fifth Dimension out of my mind... Up, up and away, in my beautiful balloon!

> *"Sing and make music in your heart to the Lord."*
> Ephesians 5:19

Now I just have to settle in and wait until the dust settles after my chemo is finished and I'm healthy enough to have the expander exchanged for the permanent implant and pump up the flat tire on the other side. So, in the meantime, if you see me veering off to the right, it's because my tires are not aligned and balanced. Just straighten me out and send me on my way again.

> *"Let your eyes look straight ahead, fix your gaze directly before you. Make level paths for your feet and take only ways that are firm. Do not swerve to the right or the left."* Proverbs 4:25-27

Hi Ho Silver, Chemo-sabi! (9/28/11)

We just returned from Dr. H's office and she wants to start my chemo treatments as soon as I get my port "installed". So, it looks like chemical warfare will begin next week sometime.

"The LORD is my strength and my song; He is my God, and I will praise Him. The LORD is a warrior; Your right hand, O LORD, shattered the enemy." Exodus 15:2-6

From now on I'm just going to say chemo, even though it will include the Herceptin and Femara (anti-estrogen). I will take the chemo & Herceptin intravenously for 18 weeks (six doses at three week intervals), then continue with the Herceptin for a year (still intravenously) as well as the Femara for five years in pill form!

I am certainly not looking forward to any of this, but Miss Fullcharge here is ready to get on with it so it will be in the rear-view mirror sooner rather than later. Thanks for all your continued prayers!

"Each pursues [her] own course like a horse charging into battle." Jeremiah 8:6

What's Not to Love About This Dead Beat Chick?! (9/30/11)

Well, I have some of a dead person's breast tissue, now I have a piece of a dead person's jaw bone from my tooth extraction today, most of my cells will be dead in a few weeks, and I will be a dead head (chemo brain). I never thought I'd be a member of the Grateful Dead! Yes, even with all this junk going on in my body, I *am* the most grateful girl around. God has blessed me beyond measure and I feel His presence with me at all times.

"...that He might be the Lord of both the dead and the living." Romans 14:9

Pink Bra Team Alert!!! (10/3/11)

It's time to rev up the **Pink Bra Team** into high gear again! For those of you who are new, I call all of you who are praying for me the **Pink Bra Team** because you lift me up, you support me so well and my cup runneth over with joy that so many of you have entered into this fight with me through your prayers. So strap yourself in because we're all in for a spiritual battle that can *only* be won through prayer!

I was just scheduled to begin my first chemo treatment on Monday, October 10th. In this next week though, I have to get my port put in (talk about a port in the storm). I'm looking at this chemo like cleaning out our house when we moved this spring. It's gonna get rid of all the junk that's collected over these 50 years in my body. You know, like all of those crazy, wacked out, mutant Diet Coke cells. I figure if my body has survived Diet Coke (and yes, TAB, in the old days!) for 45 years straight, it can handle chemotherapy. Don't I sound brave and confident *BEFORE* even getting my first treatment!?! HA!

"She has gotten so PORTly!" (10/6/11)

This is too good to not pass on to you. Do you know that you have to get a prescription from your oncologist to file with the insurance company if you need to get a cranial prosthesis? Oh, in the real world that is called a **WIG**! Ha! I crack up every time I even think of a *cranial prosthesis*! But, then I die inside thinking about going bald *myself* and actually having to wear one... and soon! They say most of the hair goes in the second week. So, unless I shave it, I'll look like Gollum from Lord of the Rings! (For those of you who haven't seen the movie, he has about six long stringy hairs on his head!! Sa-weet!)

> *"I tell you, my friends, do not be afraid of those who kill the body and after that can do no more (chemo)... Indeed, the very hairs of your head are all numbered. Don't be afraid; you are worth more than many sparrows."* Luke 12:4,7

I will be **port**-able tomorrow. I've had more unwanted poking and prodding in my body this past four months than I've have in my entire adult life!

I read that the chemo gives you a real metallic taste, so everything tastes different and mostly awful. Panic struck and I bought a mini-cake with buttercream frosting and ate the whole thing! I'm going out on a sugar high! Aaaaand, we find another meaning for the phrase, "She has gotten so portly!"

> *"How sweet are Your words to my taste, sweeter than honey to my mouth!"* Psalm 119:103

VIP ~ Veinously Implanted Port (10/9/11)

I am im**port**ant now. The surgery went well to install my port and I'm just a little tender still... just in time to get poison jammed into it! UGH! I even stayed awake through the entire Chemo Training Class. It was hard, but I did it. I wish I *had* slept through some of the side effects listings. YIKES! I pray that I don't have many of them at all.

I had to laugh; today I started packing my bag to go to the infusion center tomorrow. It was like packing a maternity bag! The funny part is that I gave birth to Brandon in less time than I will be in that chair getting my chemo tomorrow! I brought life out of one, and now this will bring death to my body...only temporarily though (I hope!!!!). In the end, life will spring up again!

> *"...rather offer yourselves to God, as those who have been brought from death to life; and offer the parts of your body to Him as instruments of righteousness."* Romans 6:13

It will take six hours for the first treatment because they have to go real slow to make sure I don't have any bad reactions. I haven't sat still that long in my adult life! We are going into totally uncharted waters tomorrow!

> *"In the end it bites like a snake and poisons like a viper. Your eyes will see strange sights and your mind imagine confusing things."* Proverbs 23:32-33

(Wow, even the Bible talks about chemo brain!)

Okay, some guys are uncomfortable being on the Pink Bra Team, so you can be on the Pink Jock Team. Even all the NFL players are wearing pink this month, so you can man-up with them!

Please pray that I will tolerate the chemo well, that I will have miraculously few side effects and can have a relatively "normal" life as I'm traveling this strange road.

> *"I lift my eyes to the hills ~ where does my help come from? My help comes from the LORD, the Maker of heaven and earth. He will not let your foot slip ~ He who watches over you will not slumber... The LORD will keep you from all harm ~ He will watch over your*

life; the LORD will watch over your coming and going both now and forevermore." Psalm 121:1-8

One Down, Five to Go! (10/10/11)

I did great today! No reactions, no nausea at all. The only thing was that they gave me a whopping dose of Benedryl® and it knocked me out for an hour and a half! At least it made the time pass quickly!!

They told me my next infusion will be Monday, October 31st. How appropriate, Halloween. They'll stir up their witch's brew and I'll transform into a zombie from Night of the Living Dead!

Wiggin' Out! (10/14/11)

Well, it's definitely feeling more real now... as in real bad. I'm already feeling weak and I'm not even in the second week where I'm REALLY supposed to feel bad. Hmmmm. It took all my energy just walking to the end of the driveway and back!

"The spirit is willing, but the body is weak." Mark 14:38

They tell me I'll lose my hair sometime next week. YIKES!

"But not a hair of your head will perish (it will just disappear for a while). By standing firm you will gain life." Luke 21:18

Gold Stars & Pink Bras (10/17/11)

I don't want to brag, buuuut... I went for my first blood work check-up this morning and that Nuelasta shot worked like crazy! Normal white blood cell counts are between 4,000 and 12,000 and mine were 27,000! I always have been an over-achiever!

I am feeling much better in the past two days than I did last week... and this is the week that I'm supposed to feel the worst. I never have been able to follow the rules very well!

"A cheerful heart is good medicine." Proverbs 17:22

Yesterday my church friends gave me a wonderful prayer shower. They put on a skit starring the church ladies (minus one, me!) and ended up stripping down to just their pink bras. Just kidding; just making sure you're not falling asleep! But, I did get my own pink bra as the leader of the Pink Bra Team. And, no I will NOT be modeling it! If you think chemo can make you sick, that would certainly do it!!

But mostly, the prayers and cards of encouragement were the most precious to me. What an incredible blessing to have such friends and sisters-in-Christ!!!!!

"Dear friends, since God so loved us, we also ought to love one another. No one has ever seen God; but if we love one another, God lives in us and His love is made complete in us. We love because He first loved us." 1 John 4:11,12,19

Coughing Up a Hairball (10/18/11)

Oh, boy! I really did it this time! I cut my hair REAL short yesterday before it comes out in long clumps in the next couple of weeks. I just thought this would be easier to see go into the trash than the long locks, but even Tinkerbell would look at my haircut and say, "Whoa! *That's* short, girl!" I think I had more hair at birth! I'm pretty sure Don can hardly wait for me to have to wear my wigs! Well, at least I won't be so sad when I go bald. Why couldn't this have happened during the heat of the summer?! It would've felt really good.

> *"Cut off your hair and throw it away; take up a lament on the barren heights."* Jeremiah 7:29

(The barren heights is now my head!)

So far so good. I've had three days where I've felt almost normal. Many would say I haven't been normal in years!!!! Maybe there *is* an upside to all of this after all!

> *"I pray that you may enjoy good health and that all may go well with you, even as your soul is getting along well."* 3 John 1:2

It's HAIRmegeddon! (10/26/11)

It must be a full moon because the wolfman, or wolfwoman, came out of nowhere this morning. I was washing my hair and I looked down at my hands and they were covered with hair!!! *Then* I got out of the shower and my shoulders and back were all hairy, too. So scary! Ow-woooooooo!

I learned the art of a good comb-over this morning. I could cover all the bald spots today, but I think this will be the last day for that. Looks like my concern about what to do about the few additional grey hairs this year and the fact that my hair is thinner than it used to be has become a moot point! See, God takes care of everything. Not the way **we** would like to see them handled every time, but...

"If a woman does not cover her head, she should have her hair cut off; and if it is a disgrace for a woman to have her hair cut or shaved off, she should cover her head." 1 Corinthians 11:6

"Remember Your word to Your servant, for You have given me hope. My comfort in my suffering is this: Your promise preserves my life. May Your unfailing love be my comfort, according to Your promise to Your servant." Psalm 119:49,50,76

Get the Rogaine Quick!!! (11/1/11)

Chemo treatment #2 is now in enemy territory on its seek and destroy mission. Feeling pretty good so far. I just got my Nuelasta shot this afternoon, so we'll see if that makes me weak again. Hmmm, my hair is almost gone and I feel weak. Samson had that same problem!

"Those who wage war against you will be nothing at all. For I am the LORD, your God, who takes hold of your right hand and says to you, Do not fear; I will help you." Isaiah 41:12-13

I decided not to shave my head. Being the nerd that I am, I see it as a science experiment. I'm kind of fascinated by the whole process. I know that's weird and that I should've just kept that to myself, but it's just part of this crazy new adventure I'm on. With the hair that I've lost so far I could make my own Chia Pet.

Hair Today, Gone Tomorrow (11/7/11)

Today was my weekly blood test and my white cell count wasn't as stellar as last month after the Nuelasta shot, but still above normal. The shot makes the bone marrow shift into overdrive to boost your germ-fighting capability, so the higher it is, the better. The nurse said that each month will vary, but it never gets up to the same level as the previous month. By January I might be a walking Petri dish, full of all kinds of creepy stuff... but hopefully none of them will be cancer cells!!

> *"[her] body well nourished, [her] bones rich with marrow."* Job 21:24

Now I know how hard it is on men when they are going bald. There's nothing you can do about it...but at least I can wear a cute hat or wig and it's only temporary for me. Another blessing to thank God for!

> *"Therefore we do not lose heart (just hair). Though outwardly we are wasting away, yet inwardly we are being renewed day by day. For our light and momentary troubles are achieving for us an eternal glory that far outweighs them all. So we fix our eyes not on what is seen, but on what is unseen. For what is seen is temporary, but what is unseen is eternal."* 2 Corinthians 4:16-18

'Leave' My Hair Alone (11/15/11)

When I woke up the other morning, I looked out at our beautiful wooded lot with the smooth lake in the background and just started to laugh. I thought "my hair is like this scene; the leaves are falling faster than you can count, and, every time the wind blows (aka: when I use the hair blower) they come off even faster and just swirl around until they fall to the ground. What's left of the view is a smooth, glistening white surface and a few straggler leaves clinging for dear life!"

"You will be like an oak with fading leaves." Isaiah 1:30

"Make yourselves as bald as the vulture." Micah 1:16

More good results from my blood work today. Everything is still in the normal range.

All in all, I count myself one of the most blessed women on the planet! Just thinking about Thanksgiving makes me more and more thankful all the time. I'm especially thankful for my new turkey breast and its stuffing!

"From them will come songs of thanksgiving and the sound of rejoicing." Jeremiah 30:19

"And we pray this in order that you may live a life worthy of the Lord and may please Him in every way: bearing fruit in every good work, growing in the knowledge of God, being strengthened with all power according to His glorious might so that you may have great endurance and patience, and joyfully giving thanks to the Father, Who has qualified you to share in the inheritance of the saints in the kingdom of light." Colossians 1:10-12

Brandon sent me this pin. I love it!

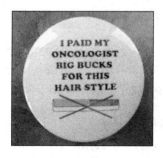

True or False? (11/18/11)

False: Boob

False: Tooth

False: Hair

True: My love for Jesus and all of you!!!

"You were taught,...to put off your old self,...and to put on the new self, created to be like God in true righteousness and holiness." Ephesians 4:22-24

Thought you might like to see the new "Cranial Prosthesis" (aka - my wig) that I'm sporting.

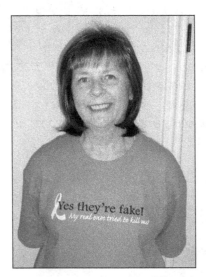

Sometimes I have to smile when I read in the Psalms:

*"...in God I trust; I will not be afraid. What **can man do to me?**"* Psalm 56:10-12

*"The Lord is with me; I will not be afraid. What **can man do to me?**"* Psalm 118:5-7

*"So we say with confidence, "The Lord is my helper; I will not be afraid. What **can man do to me?**"* Hebrews 13:5-7

Well, actually, man can do *a lot* to me!!!! Going through cancer treatment is hard on the body, hard on the emotions, hard to stay mentally "up" for the next step into the unknown, and sometimes hard spiritually to claim the promises of God when you feel terrible or test results take a turn for the worse. But I believe with all my heart that it's all in your perspective. Or, should I say, God's perspective.

If you aren't real familiar with your Bible and don't know where to find promise after promise in His Word, go buy a book of God's Promises. Read them over and over, memorize key passages that hold special meaning for you, hide them in your heart and mind so that when you become fearful or discouraged, you can pull them out and claim them! Remember, we are **more** than conquerors in Christ Jesus! What can man do to me? Lots. What can Jesus do to me? More than we can ask or imagine!

> *"What, then, shall we say in response to this? If God is for us, who can be against us?"* Romans 8:30-32

> *"Do not be afraid of those who kill the body but cannot kill the soul."* Matthew 10:27

> *"Jesus Christ heals you."* Acts 9:33-35

> *"Therefore we do not lose heart. Though outwardly we are wasting away, yet inwardly we are being renewed day by day. For our light and momentary trouble are achieving for us an eternal glory that far outweighs them all. So we fix our eyes not on what is seen, but on what is unseen. For what is seen is temporary, but what is unseen is eternal."* 2 Corinthians 4:16-18

~6~

UNEXPECTED BLESSINGS ABOUND!

God bREaST Ye Merry, Gentlemen (12/9/11)

It's The Most Wonderful Time of The Year!

I love decorating for Christmas! Our 10' tall Christmas tree looks so beautiful in our new house. Well, I too have a brand new handmade Christmas ornament perched high on my tree this year! Unfortunately chemo halted the progress on my reconstruction project, so I will have to wait until summer to have a new pair of jingle bells.

> *"The women are...tripping along...with ornaments jingling. Therefore the LORD will bring sores on the heads of the women; the LORD will make their scalps bald."* Isaiah 3:16-17

Good thing it's not about *me* this Christmas, but it's **all** about Jesus. Even with all of our trials and imperfect situations, we can still rejoice and give thanks to The One who came to earth to make us spiritually whole and reconciles us with the Father. Someday Jesus will return and our bodies will also be whole and we will be made perfect.

"The Son is the radiance of God's glory and the exact representation of His being." Hebrews 1:3

It truly is the most wonderful time of the year (aside from Easter). Let's all make like Christmas trees; shine brightly for Christ, bring joy to all who see us, and give the gift of love to those who really need it!

"It is more blessed to give than to receive." Acts 20:35

On The Fourth Round of Chemo My True Love Gave to Me... (12/17/11)

Well, darn; I'm not invincible after all. This fourth chemo treatment has kicked my butt. The first week after my infusion is always the toughest, but this past week was my weakest and most sore yet. I've been rotating the heating pad on every part of my body except my head, probably because there is hardly any hair or brain function left to bother with!

"The vigor of [her] step is weakened...I will boast all the more gladly about my weaknesses, so that Christ's power may rest on me...For when I am weak, then I am strong...Therefore, strengthen your feeble arms and weak knees...so that the lame may not be disabled, but rather healed." Job 18:7, 2 Cor. 12:9-10, Hebrews 12:12

We're praying hard that the next two weeks will be as good as they have been the last three treatments.

"But for you who revere My name, the sun of righteousness will rise with healing in its wings. And you will go out and leap like calves released from the stall." Malachi 4:2

"How can we thank God enough for you in return for all the joy we have in the presence of our God because of you?" 1 Thessalonians 3:9

Our greatest "presence" this year are the gifts of family and friends loving on us so well and the most precious gift of all; Jesus coming to earth to give us *"the life that is truly life."* 1 Timothy 6:19

"But the angel said to them, 'Do not be afraid, I bring you good news of great joy that will be for all the people.'" Luke 2:10

One of my favorite Christmas songs since I was a child has a verse in it that often comes to mind when things aren't going like I'd hoped. It says, "And when you're worried and you can't sleep, count your blessings instead of sheep, and you'll fall asleep, counting your blessings." I'm an optimist at heart, but sometimes we all have to really dig to think of a blessing in the midst of our mess. I think that's what David had in mind when he wrote Psalm 9:1-2. He was in the middle of a fight for his very life as his enemies hunted him down.

"I will give thanks to the Lord with my whole heart; I will recount all of Your wonderful deeds. I will be glad and exult in You; I will sing praise to Your name, O Most High."

If we recount all the times God has been faithful and good to us, it changes our outlook. We are prone to think "I'm the only one this has happened to. Nobody else can relate. I'm in this alone." We *know* in our minds that it isn't true, but we still sink down in that pit...even feeling abandoned by God at times. That's the most important time to list God's attributes. When you fall into the pit, the only light you can see comes from above. The Apostle Paul knew well what it was like to face severe trials of all types, yet he says in Philippians 4:8,

"Whatever is true, whatever is noble, whatever is right, whatever is pure, whatever is lovely, whatever is admirable-if anything is excellent or praiseworthy-think about such things."

Can You Hear Me Now?! (1/3/12)

I'm scheduled to have my 5th chemo treatment. They can't do it if my white blood cell count is too low. My first blood test last time was enormous at 23,000, but the following week it had dropped like a rock to only 4,300.

I started the morning with a very ominous sign; there were 10 vultures perched in our trees right outside the bathroom window. I'm not exaggerating, 10!! But I just looked at them in the meanest look I could muster and said, "Not today, you ole buzzards, not today!" Okay, that was an exaggeration; I didn't say that at all. I didn't even think it until now, but it does add flair to the story.

"Wherever there is a carcass, there the vultures will gather." Matthew 24:28

Oooh, it was a close call. My numbers were right at the cut-off (3,100). Whew! So I was able to get my chemo treatment. Seriously, how twisted is that when you're excited about chemo. Just that I only have one more treatment to go now!!!!!!!!!!!!!!!!!!!!!! Yee Haw! I still will have to go in every three weeks until the end of the year for my Herceptin infusion, but that will only take an hour, not six.

I think you all crashed the system in heaven there was so much activity all at once. Go Prayer Warriors!! You're the best! Just think, most of us (I'm praying for ALL) will get to spend the rest of eternity together! Now there's a HugFest I'm thrilled to be a part of!!!

"On Him we have set our hope that He will continue to deliver us, as you help us by your prayers. Then many will give thanks on our behalf for the gracious favor granted us in answer to the prayers of many." 2 Corinthians 1:10-11

One Blessing After Another! (1/4/12)

I was struck today (it didn't hurt though!) when I was talking to someone about how many ways God has mani-fested Himself in my life through my cancer. I know this will sound weird, but I have never felt as joyful and exhilarated as I have been through this whole ordeal. I have seen God break down barriers, change hearts, renew relationships and countless other things that could've only happened through my situation. Things that seemed impossible to me, God has made a way and has blessed me beyond my wildest imagi-nation. Nobody wants cancer, but it has been the biggest blessing in so many ways that I thank God for it.

"Let us run with perseverance the race marked out for us. Let us fix our eyes on Jesus, the author and perfecter of our faith, who for the joy set before Him endured the cross..." Hebrews 12:1-2

Please don't misunderstand me, I am not equating my cancer to Christ's crucifixion by any stretch, but just pointing to the fact that Jesus looked past the cross and endured the excruciating temporary pain because He could see in His mind returning to His rightful heavenly home in full glory. Lord willing, I will be over and done with this mess soon and I look forward with excitement to what He has for me on the other side! More joy inexpressible!

"Behold, I make all things new... Write, for these words are true and faithful." Revelation 21:5

Did Anyone Get Their License Plate?! (1/9/12)

The last thing I remember seeing was the underbelly of the 18-wheeler that ran over me last week. Then, they backed up to run me over again and off they went on their merry way, leaving me in the dust. Well, at least that's what it felt like this week after my 5th chemo treatment & Nuelasta shot. It's a good thing I only have one more to go. Yea!!!!!!!!!!!!!!!!!!!!!!!!!!!

"Be merciful to me, LORD, for I am faint; O LORD, heal me, for my bones are in agony." Psalm 6:2

My white blood cell count was only 12,600 today. That's still just over the normal range, but last time it was 23,000, so I don't have much room for it to drop in the next two weeks. The crummy part is that there really isn't anything you can do to boost it. Trust me; I've gone online to check. I'd even give up my Diet Coke if that would work...NOT! Well, maybe temporarily.

"He will rescue them...for precious is their blood in His sight." Psalm 72:14

"But let all who take refuge in You be glad; let them ever sing for joy. Spread Your protection over them that those who love Your name may rejoice in You. For surely, O LORD, you bless the righteous; You surround them with Your favor as with a shield." Psalm 5:11-12

Calling For an Up-rising...of My White Blood Cells (1/16/12)

"For the eyes of the LORD range throughout the earth to strengthen those whose hearts are fully committed to Him." 2 Chronicles 16:9

I'm right here, Lord! I need You to strengthen my white blood cells! Will You please do an "increase and multiply" command to my WBC!?! You've already done that with my fat cells without me even asking!! UGH!

My WBC count this morning was only 3,600... with a week to go. More and fervent prayer please!!!

"I am bowed down and brought very low." Psalm 38:6

(Thankfully, that only refers to my WB cells, not my spirit.)

I just love my doctor's staff. The gal that takes my blood every week just kept saying to me today, "Keep the faith! Just keep the faith!" God has placed believers all around me. My oncologist even gives seminars on "Faith and Your Cancer". How cool is *that*?!

"But one thing I do: Forgetting what is behind and straining toward what is ahead, I press on toward the goal to win the prize." Philippians 3:13-14

Only one more chemo treatment to go! Isn't that amazing?! I pray that there is nothing standing in the way of getting it on time. Hopefully it will be next Tuesday (not my usual Monday). Storm the gates of heaven again team and we'll all celebrate together when it is all over!!! Giant Hug-A-Thon when I recover!!!!!!!! Can't wait!

You may have heard the saying, "It's not so much *what* happens to you, but *how* you respond to it that matters." Most of the time we can't control what happens to us, but we make "fork-in-the-road" decisions every single day. And each fork sets us on a different path. Almost every one of my doctors told me, "You will do well because of your positive attitude and your strong faith." My oncologists both told me that they can just about tell who will do well and who won't when they first come in, just by their attitude.

There will be many times in your trials of life where your circumstances look overwhelming. I am always reminded of how Jesus *wants* us to handle adversity in Matthew 14:22-32...and how we all too often fall short. It is the story about Peter walking on the water with Jesus. Peter had seen Jesus do mind-boggling things, so he asked Jesus for permission to 'do the impossible' and walk with Him on the stormy sea. Even though Peter **knew** he could totally trust Jesus and *was actually walking on water along with Jesus,* he took his eyes off Jesus and could only focus on the frightening waves that sought to overtake him and plunge him into the depths... and he started sinking. The sea wasn't any stormier than when he jumped out of the boat, but he simply forgot Who controlled the waves.

The passage also says it was *"during the fourth watch of the night".* That is the darkest time. And isn't that what we often do? When things are the darkest in our trial, we take our eyes off Jesus and become "terrified" at our circumstances. We quickly sink and it feels like we are about to drown. But, like Peter did, we can snap out of it long enough to look up, reach out and call out for Jesus to save us. The passage says, **"Immediately** *Jesus reached out His hand and caught him. 'You of little faith,' He said, 'why did you doubt?'"* You see, Jesus hadn't moved, Peter's focus had...and he was rescued once again by clinging to Jesus.

Big waves look totally different to a novice surfer than they do to an experienced boarder. To one they look petrifying; to the other they look exhilarating! That's how it is with our faith and trust in the Lord. The longer we walk with Jesus and learn how trustworthy and faithful He is through personal experience over the years, the less anxious we will be when our big waves come. We don't have to be swept away by them...we can be lifted up on top of them for the ride of our lives.

> *"Fear not, for I have redeemed you; I have summoned you by name; you are mine. When you pass through the waters, **I will be with you**; and when you pass through the rivers, they will not sweep over you. When you walk through the fire, you will not be burned; the flames will not set you ablaze. For I am the LORD, your God, the Holy One of Israel, your Savior."* Isaiah 43:1-3

Let The Cell-ebrating Begin! 1/23/12

You know what they say, "Go big or go home!" Well, my WBC count wasn't big at all, in fact it was *really* low, but they didn't send me home.

"They will tell of the power of Your awesome works, and I will proclaim Your great deeds. They will celebrate Your abundant goodness and joyfully sing of Your righteousness." Psalm 145:6-7

Instead, God answered our prayers in a way that NONE of us could ever have imagined. The oncologist simply canceled my last chemo treatment! So I'm totally done with my chemo treatments!!!!!!!! She said I have done so well that we don't really need to do anymore. So now I'm just sitting here getting my Herceptin infusion. Wow!!

What an awesome God we have!!!!!

"And the God of all grace, who called you to his eternal glory in Christ, after you have suffered a little while, will Himself restore you and make you strong, firm and steadfast." 1 Peter 5:10-11

Another Hair-Raising Adventure (1/25/12)

"No eye has seen, no ear has heard, no mind has conceived what God has prepared for those who love him." 1 Corinthians 2:9

I still can't get over what God did yesterday! I already feel like I'm getting healthier!!

Well, the time has come for my science experiment with

my hair to end. I have lived with the "Linus" look (from the Peanuts comic strip) for four months and this morning I switched characters and became "Charlie Brown" (minus the one hair on his forehead). My oncologist gave me the understatement of the year when she said that my "hair would just thin out, but not all of it would fall out". She knows her business! But I decided to have Don shave it all off this morning since the new growth might start appearing in the near future and who knows in what form it will sprout!!! An older lady (77) in the infusion center yesterday told me her hair came in pitch back!! See, another science experiment for me to look forward to!!!! I can't even imagine.

"But the hair on [her] head began to grow again after it had been shaved." Judges 16:22

Here she is, the Chemo Queen!

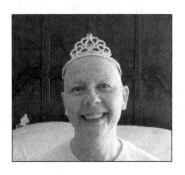

In so many ways this has been the best worst six months. For as crazy as it sounds, I wouldn't trade it for anything. I know I still have a ways to go until I'm done with everything, but I feel like I'm over the hump!

Speaking of humps... now I'm three weeks closer to getting the party started on my reconstruction! Dr. S can finish blowing up the balloon on February 14th. Life is definitely looking brighter today!

"Oh LORD my God, I called to you for help and You healed me." Psalm 30:2

Ac-CELL-erating Slowly (1/30/12)

It feels like Groundhog Day every week when I go get my blood work. I pop my head out and see whether I have to get back in my burrow for another week, or, if I can start venturing out basking in the sunshine again with the rest of the world. Instead of Punxatawney Phil, I'm Chemo Karen.

Well, winter's not over yet and I have to stay in hibernation for a while longer; my WBCs have only risen from 2500 last week to 3300 this week. Still not in the normal range (4000-12000). The WBCs don't make you feel any better or worse; they are the infection fighters. So, even though I feel fine, my insides are telling me I'm not yet strong enough to emcee my Hug-A-Thon yet. DARN!

"Let them rise up to help you!" Deuteronomy 32:38

"Rise to my defense!" Psalm 35:23

"Long life to you! Good health to you and your household! And good health to all that is yours!" 1 Samuel 25:5-7

If I Didn't Have Random Thoughts, It Would Be a Pretty Lonely Place Under My Wig!! (2/3/12)

I had one of those random thoughts today (like most every day!). Back in the day, there was a toy called Weebles (Google it!). They were little rolly-poly things, bottom-heavy, with smiling faces. Hmmmm, sounds way too much like me! The tag line for them said, "Weebles Wobble, but they don't fall down." Wouldn't it be wonderful if all of us could be Weeble Christians! There are so many things in this life that send us wobbling, but if we trust in Jesus He won't let us fall down.

"If the LORD delights in a man's way, He makes his steps firm; though he stumble, he will not fall, for the LORD upholds him with His hand." Psalm 37:23-24

That's how I've felt during this whole cancer process. Stuff like that certainly rocks your world, but we have a God that holds us up in the midst of the wobbly times. He promises to never leave us or forsake us and we can claim that *"in ALL things God works for the good of those who love Him"*. Now that's a random thought to take hold of and never let go of!!!!

Saline, Saline, Over the Ocean Blue (2/14/12)

Now where were we before I was so rudely interrupted by chemotherapy? Yeees, that's right, we were talking about getting cuter hooters way back in September. So let's start talking about the exciting stuff again!!

"Your breasts were formed and your hair grew." Ezekiel 16:7

I have taken up saline as my new hobby. This morning I loaded up my 'saline vessel', the Love Boat, and I'm ship-shape now. I shall now be called Captain Karen. Since I already have a 'port', I cruised to get my blood test (Yea! It was 4,900. Finally in the hugging range!!) and Herceptin infusion this afternoon. If that isn't a romantic Valentine's Day, I don't know what is. BUT, it gets me closer to my final destination, so that *IS* a sweet treat and I will treasure it in my heart (or, at least near my heart) forever!

"Then they cried out to the LORD in their trouble, and He brought them out of their distress. He stilled the storm to a whisper; the waves of the sea were hushed. They were glad when it grew calm, and He

guided them to their desired haven. Let them give
thanks to the LORD for His unfailing love and His
wonderful deeds."* Psalm 107:28-31

Full speed ahead, Captain!! Hoooooot! Hoooter!

"Love one another deeply, from the heart." 1 Peter 1:22

SPRING IS IN THE hAIR! (3/6/12)

Cha-cha-cha-chia! Oh, yes, I'm in early-stage Chia Pet
mode now! My hair is about ¼ inch long now and so far real
dark... except a few totally white hairs! YIKES! Too early to
tell what texture it will be though. Stay tuned...

*"And do not swear by your head, for you cannot
make even one hair white or black."* Matthew 5:36

The other thing that's growing is my white blood cell
number. Today it was 7,800... right in the middle of the
normal range!

And, to top off the springy, growy theme: This weekend
we went to see Brandon and Jenn and the twins in TX. The
boys are 2½ now and they have been trying to get them
to say Grammy with no success. Instead, in the moment
Christian called me 'Garden'!!! Who knows how that came
about, but it sure was cute hearing him say it!!

"No tree in the garden of God could match its beauty."
Ezekiel 31:8

Sailing, Saline... (5/27/12)

Well, I took another big step this week; I went out in public
without my wig or a hat!!! Just in time for the hot summer!

There were a few double-takes, but no gasps, so that was encouraging! It's not long enough to know if it will be curly yet, but it has blondish highlights in it (against the usual brown backdrop). I've always wanted highlights, but was never willing to pay for it, so God blessed me with one of the "desires of my heart". That's just like Him to delight in giving us even silly things like that!!

> *"The wilderness will rejoice and blossom. Like the crocus; it will burst into bloom; it will rejoice greatly and shout for joy."* Isaiah 35:1-2

We are heading off on our big cruise on Tuesday. We planned it to celebrate my post-chemo (and hopefully post-cancer forever!), as well as pre-reconstruction. When I get home it will be time to put on my pink hard hat again because we are putting the finishing touches on the temple! It will have two well-built arches placed right out front with salt-water pools under them. It will be so nice to get this finished. I was hoping my theme song could be "June is *Bust*in' Out All Over", but I couldn't get it scheduled until early July (I'll let you know when to start praying again once I get the schedule), so I'll have to come up with a new song.

"Sing to the LORD, for He has done glorious things; let this be known to all the world. Shout aloud and sing for joy!" Isaiah 12:5-6

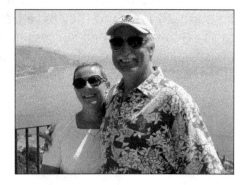

~7~

ON TO BIGGER & BETTER THINGS!

I'm Starting a New Job Soon! (7/3/12)

H a! I bet that was more shocking news than when I told you I had breast cancer! But, you can put your minds to rest because Princesses don't get *real* jobs, we just get boob jobs.

The surgeon just called and they have scheduled my reconstruction surgery for THIS Monday, July 9th, at 10:30am.

"Like cold water to a thirsty soul, so is good news from a distant land." Proverbs 25:25

I'm really excited to get this done. I feel like I will be "over the hump" once this is completed. The worst part of this past six months has been simply *waiting* to get back to "normal" from the chemo... especially since I felt back to normal almost immediately. I'm the kind of person that just wants to get it over and done with sooner rather than later, so I'm *reeeeeally* ready to get this behind me... or should I say, in front of me.

Please pray that everything goes smoothly and that I will heal up quickly. Thanks Pink Bra (and Jock) Team!!!! You're the breast!

"The LORD has done great things for us, and we are filled with joy" **...and saline!** Psalm 126:3

What's the Breakfast Special of the Day? *(7/9/12)*

2 EGGS SUNNYSIDE UP, COMIN' RIGHT UP!

Well, it's almost time for the final phase of the temple construction. Don't expect anything monumental though; in tough economic times like these, a small fortune doesn't buy Solomon's Temple anymore. You'll probably wonder what all the hoopla has been about this past year, but I'm going for quality, not quantity. Maybe "chapel" would be a more fitting term.

"In Him the whole building is joined together and rises to become a holy temple in the Lord." Ephesians 2:21

My surgery is at 10:30am. I will be staying one night in the Cone Day Surgery Center (isn't that an oxymoron?!). Please pray that Dr. S (plastic surgeon) will have no problems with the surgery and that I "bounce" back quickly from this surgery. I have grandtwins to see this summer!!! Don will send out an update later in the day.

"Fashion a breastpiece...the work of a skilled craftsman." Exodus 28:15

I'm thinking about releasing a new CD when I recover from all this. I'll call it "TREASURE CHEST: The BrEaST Uplifting Songs of Our Time". Some of the songs will include: "You Raise

Me Up", "Your Love's Liftin' Me Higher Than I've Ever Been Lifted Before", "Mamories", "I Want To Take You Higher", "Up, Up and Away In My Beautiful Balloon", "Ain't No Mountain High Enough", and "I've Got You Under My Skin". In keeping with my reconstructive surgery, I am offering a "buy one, get one free" package. This is for a limited time only, so act now!

"In His love and mercy He redeemed them; He lifted them up." Isaiah 63:9

"The Lord upholds all who are falling and raises up all who are bowed down." Psalm 145:14

I'm Doing the BrEaST I Can Under the Circumstances (7/12/12)

My theme song for this week is "Love Me Tender". Ouch!

"And the God of all grace, who called you to His eternal glory in Christ, after you have suffered a little while, will Himself restore you and make you strong, firm and steadfast." 1 Peter 5:10

I've done really well so far... thanks to my two bosom buddies Vicoden and Valium! I started "weaning" myself off the Vicoden today and haven't felt bad, so that's good!

Thanks for all your prayers and notes! It's been quite a year, but now on to bigger and better things!

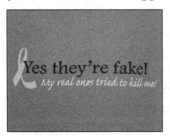
Yes they're fake!
My real ones tried to kill me!

"When all the people saw [her]...praising God...at the temple gate called Beautiful, they were filled with wonder and amazement at what had happened to [her]". Acts 3:9-1

The Finishing Touches (7/18/12)

As I write what I hope is the final entry in this chapter of my life, I am overwhelmed with gratitude for all of you who have stood by me in so many ways... but most especially for storming the gates of heaven on my behalf so many times. That is a true gift of God and I will forever treasure each one of you for lifting me up. How many times did we all see Him answer our prayers in such unique ways?!

"No eye has seen, no ear has heard, no mind has conceived what God has prepared for those who love Him." 1 Corinthians 2:9

I'm healing up well. I still have a few minor procedures to finish up by the end of the year, but let's just leave it at that, I still have to install the "dome of the rock" later this year (sorry to mix religions here, but it *is* on the temple mount!). You won't be hearing more about that, rest assured.

This cancer journey reminds me of the story of how a pearl is formed. The poor little lowly oyster just hums along trying to avoid becoming oysters on the half shell or Oysters Rockefeller when someone kicks sand in her face. She shakes it off, but one tiny grain of sand gets lodged inside her. It becomes an irritant and her body tries to eradicate it by putting layer upon layer of "boo-boo cream" on it. Over time that initial "injury" becomes a beautiful pearl. It was the suffering and struggle that culminated in something much more valuable than ever imagined. So, the important take-away from that little parable is that I now have two pearls of great price!!! WooHoo!

"Again, the kingdom of heaven is like a merchant seeking beautiful pearls, who, when he had found

one pearl of great price, went and sold all that he had and bought it." Matthew 13:44-45

As I've said before, no one ever wants hardships like cancer in their lives, but if this breast cancer is what it took to grow my faith to what it is today, know the Lord in a much deeper way, to watch the body of Christ be who God intended them to be, and to view the Kingdom of God with a more realistic, heavenly perspective... then I gratefully accept it and even cherish it. I know I can trust that whatever He allows in my life is there to draw me closer to Him and make me more like Jesus every day (oh boy, now that's a miracle of all miracles!). If I was given the choice to turn back the clock and skip this year, I wouldn't. God has made me clear out a lot of "stuff" in my life the past several years, but it was so He would feel more at home in my heart. (I didn't know He was going to clear out a whole breast to make a little salt-water pond in His newly renovated home though!). But now He has a bit more elbow room to work in me and through me.

"But the pot He was shaping from the clay was marred in his hands; so the Potter formed it into another pot, shaping it as seemed best to Him." Jeremiah 18:4

"But blessed is the [wo]man who trusts in the LORD, whose confidence is in Him. [S]he will be like a tree planted by the water that sends out its roots by the stream. It does not fear when heat comes; its leaves are always green. It has no worries in a year of drought and never fails to bear fruit." Jeremiah 17:7-8

I've Been Busted! (11/11/12)

Well, just when you thought I was done writing to you, *surprise*! Please pray for me tomorrow morning as I go into my last surgery (hopefully!).

It is time to put the finishing touches on, but I decided to change plastic surgeons for the last step in my temple reconstruction and she's not a fan of saline, so she's going to do some more slicing and dicing and put in silicone. So, from now on I will be referring to my cleavage as my own personal Silicone Valley.

> *"I went...to look at the new growth in the valley."*
> Song of Solomon 6:1

So this little turkey will have new stuffing for Thanksgiving (it won't be nearly as salty). And I **am** *very* thankful that this is the last surgery!!!! Well, I do have to get de-port-ed in December, but they said that will be a breeze. The oncologist wants to hold off taking my port out until my last CT Scan results come back.

> *"Come out of her...Give back to her as she has given;
> ...a double portion from her own <u>cup</u>."* Revelation 18:6

> *"Since we are receiving a kingdom that cannot be shaken, let us be thankful."* Hebrews 12:28

Jingle All the Way! (12/19/12)

All I can say is "I am going to be really ticked if the Mayan calendar is right and we're toast this Friday after all I've been through this past year and a half!" But at least I'll go out as a bombshell bursting in air!

Truly though, I am in God's hands no matter what day it is and what happens on any given day. What a comfort that has been over the course of this cancer journey. I think this portion of Psalm 73 sums up my relationship with the Lord:

"Nevertheless, I am continually with You; You hold my right hand. You guide me with Your counsel, and afterward You will receive me to glory. Whom have I in heaven but You? And there is nothing on earth that I desire besides You. My flesh and my heart may fail but God is the strength of my heart and my portion forever. But for me it is good to be near God. I have made the Lord God my refuge, that I may tell of all Your works." Psalm 73:25,26,28

I am dearly de-port-ed now, so I'm officially ALL DONE!

"Better is the end of a thing than its beginning." Ecclesiastes 4:8

So to "recap" the last year and a half, (a definite pun intended), I've had two breast implants (actually four counting the "redo"!) and three tooth implants, but most important of all, I have Jesus deeply implanted in my heart.

"For whoever has despised the day of small things shall rejoice." Zechariah 4:10

I'm so looking forward to 2013 being the beginning of a new era of just a few check-ups here and there... all ending with "You're doing great!" But at least I won the *booby* prize for most doctors' appointments in one year at 91, so I'm happy!

Merry Christmas to all you of on my Pink Bra Team! I am so grateful to you all! But most of all, I'm forever grateful to God for giving us the ultimate present, His "presence" through Jesus Christ, our Lord, on a Christmas long ago... and every day since then. Eternal life; the only gift that lasts forever and never wears out... in fact, it gets more precious with age!

"And she whistled, & shouted, & called them by name!

Now Slasher, now Cancer, now Prance like a Vixen

(Hey, I have to show off my new cuter hooters!),

On Vomit, on Stupid (chemo brain!), on-Cologist Blitzen.

Now slash away! Slash away! Slash away all!"

Many breast cancer races give you the option to run in someone's name. Several people last year told me they were running/walking for me (along with many other women they knew who have either succumbed to the disease or have become "survivors" in their fight).

Well, we are all in the race of our lives...our eternal lives. The author of Hebrews wrote,

> *"Therefore we also, since we are surrounded by so great a cloud of witnesses, let us throw off everything that hinders and the sin that so easily entangles, and let us run with perseverance the race marked out for us. Let us fix our eyes on Jesus... so that you will not grow weary and lose heart."* Hebrews 12:1-3

We are running the race in honor of Jesus. He claimed ultimate victory over death and the horrible disease of sin. Since He died that we might live, let each one of us live (run) like the gold medal winners that we truly are, so when we hit the finish line we will hear *"Well done, good and faithful servant! Come and share in your Master's happiness!"* (Matthew 25:21)

I'd like to end this book with some Scripture as an encouragement for you to **Press On** to the finish line!

"But one thing I do: Forgetting what is behind and straining toward what is ahead, I press on toward the goal to win the prize." Philippians 3:13-14

"But we also rejoice in our sufferings, because we know that suffering produces perseverance; perseverance, character; and character, hope. And hope does not disappoint us, because God has poured out His love into our hearts by the Holy Spirit, whom He has given us." Romans 5:3-5

"Consider it pure joy, my brothers (and sisters), whenever you face trials of many kinds, because you know that the testing of your faith develops perseverance. Perseverance must finish its work so that you may be mature and complete, not lacking anything." James 1:2-4

"...we have this hope as an anchor for the soul, firm and secure... Let us hold unswervingly to the hope we profess, for He who promised is faithful." Hebrews 6:19, 10:23

"He gives strength to the weary and increases the power of the weak." Isaiah 40:29

"For I am the LORD, your God, who takes hold of your right hand and says to you, Do not fear; I will help you." Isaiah 41:13

"Have I not commanded you? Be strong and coura-geous. Do not be terrified; do not be discouraged, for the LORD your God will be with you wherever you go." Joshua 1:9

"My flesh and my heart may fail, but God is the strength of my heart and my portion forever." Psalm 73:26

"Though outwardly we are wasting away, yet inwardly we are being renewed day by day." 2 Corinthians 4:16

"Peace I leave with you; My peace I give you. I do not give to you as the world gives. Do not let your hearts be troubled and do not be afraid." John 14:27

"You will not have to fight this battle. Take up your positions; **stand firm** and see the deliverance the Lord will give you. Do not be afraid; do not be discouraged. Go out to face them tomorrow, and the Lord will be with you." 2 Chronicles 20:16-18

"In all these things we are more than conquerors through Him who loved us. For I am convinced that neither death nor life, neither angels nor demons, neither the present nor the future, nor any powers, neither height nor depth, nor anything else in all cre-ation, will be able to separate us from the love of God that is in Christ Jesus our Lord." Romans 8 37-39

~8~

WHAT IF?

I hope I have not seemed cavalier to you throughout this book. I truly haven't meant to be! You might be thinking, "It's easy for you to sound so upbeat since you had a 'relatively mild' kind of cancer. I, on the other hand, have Stage 4 cancer and my prognosis isn't quite so clear." There may be some truth to that, but we must *choose* how to go through *each* of our trials. We can cling tightly to God, as when we are plunging straight down on a roller coaster, hanging on for dear life, or fight against God like a toddler being dragged from a toy store. One is an exhilarating wild ride, all the while our adrenaline is pumping like crazy, and the other is an exhausting, exasperating, sob-filled drama...for not just you, but everyone around you. Pastor David Jeremiah said, "... open hands—especially in the midst of a crisis—puts God first. When we give to Him with open hands, He not only blesses us but He takes what He wants and gives back what we need. Humanly speaking, it may not make sense. But put God first in your life, and watch what He will do."

Life isn't always a fairy tale with everything ending "happily ever after". It's more like "happily EVEN after" ...even after a terrifying diagnosis or less-than-optimistic prognosis ...even after harsh cancer treatments... even after the scars, both physical and emotional... even after (you fill in the blank).

Given the hand we have been dealt, let's go through some of the 'what if's' that you may be wrestling with... and some that may not have even occurred to you until now.

What *if* God actually *chose you* to bring Him glory through this cancer?

Have you asked, "Why me?!" Without sounding cold, why **not** you? God may have a uniquely special story for you to tell. Maybe the better question would be, "If me, what do You want me to learn through this?" Or, "If me, how can I lift Your name up and glorify You each day in spite of my disease?" Or, "If me, who is it that you want me to 'touch' during this time to draw into Your Kingdom?"

One of the early church fathers, Augustine, said, "Trials come to prove and improve us."

No matter what the outcome of your cancer is, you can trust that this trial has been filtered through God's hands. A godly response to your trial is quite compelling to others. You have a powerful platform to speak into the lives of people that ordinarily might not listen to you.

"For we are God's workmanship, created in Christ Jesus to do good works, which God prepared in advance for us to do." Ephesians 2:10

What *if* God allowed this into your life for His eternal purposes?

If you aren't a Christian, He may be drawing you to Himself through this trial. Our son, Brandon, had heard the Gospel message many times before, and gave intellectual ascent to it, but it wasn't until *his* cancer that he had to decide if God was *"real"* <u>to him</u> or not. God met him in his deepest need and came alive to him like never before.

Sometimes God needs to get our attention, other times He wants to cement our relationship with Him, and still others, He wants to take us to a new level of knowing and trusting Him. Any way He does it, it's all good!

"Taste and see that the LORD is good; blessed is the man who takes refuge in Him." Psalm 34:8

And, if you *are* a believer in Jesus Christ, He may be giving you the opportunity to share your faith and trust in Him in a way that you wouldn't ordinarily have been able to when you were healthy. Many of the people who followed me on my CaringBridge® site are not believers, but they observed my strong faith and the corresponding Scripture verses that had become dear to me. I grabbed hold of more and more of God's promises in His Word with each new bend in the road, even the Scriptures I occasionally took out of context in a light-hearted way.

One of my old pastors said, "The saying 'You can lead a horse to water, but you can't make him drink', isn't really true. If you give him enough salt, he'll drink." In Matthew 5:13, Jesus says, *"You are the salt of the earth. But if the salt loses its saltiness, how can it be made salty again?"* Your cancer just may draw others into a **real** relationship with the Savior and Lord of life! So don't lose your saltiness. Sprinkle it generously wherever you go!

Sometimes I think God tests us to see if we will be a 'Job' or 'Job's wife'. Job's response to their immense trial was *"Shall we accept good from God, and not trouble?"* (Job 2:10). Job's wife responded with *"Curse God and die!"*

(Job 2:9). We *say* we trust and depend on God, but it's only under the **really big trials** that our true hearts are revealed. I praise God that my testings have plunged me into an even deeper relationship withHim. I watched *Him* come through to provide all I needed when I had exhausted my best efforts.

What if God is trying to tear down a big idol of yours... or several?

Idols are simply things or people who compete with God's attention in your life. Are good health, self-sufficiency, comfort, and security some things you cling to or take pride in? I only mention those because they are issues I struggle with! Ask Him to show you *your* idols, but be forewarned; He **will** show you. Don't waste your cancer experience by not seeking God's highest for you. Allow Him to destroy those idols that have been keeping you from fully depending on Him and knowing Him at a deeper level than ever before.

> *"So I say to you: Ask and it will be given to you; seek and you will find; knock and the door will be opened to you. For everyone who asks receives; he who seeks finds; and to him who knocks, the door will be opened."* Luke 11:9-10

What if the cancer comes back?!

Several people have told me "I've survived two bouts of cancer and I'm still here!" I **know** they meant that statement as an encouragement, but it made my heart sink each time I heard it. I don't even want to think of the possibility that once I'm done with this battle that another one may be on the horizon someday.

Some people spend the rest their lives with this dark cloud hovering ominously over their heads wondering if their cancer will return. Well, if it does, we will just have to deal with it like any other bump in the road. Whether your cancer comes back or not, this won't be the last trial you will face, so we all need to treasure promises like this:

> *"We who have fled to take hold of the hope offered to us may be greatly encouraged. We have this hope as an anchor for the soul, firm and secure."* Hebrews 6:18-19

> *"Though I walk **through** the valley of the shadow of death, I will fear no evil, for You are with me."* Psalm 23:4

We are not to camp in the valley of the shadow of death, but pass through it. For many of our trials it is only a shadow, so we must not become paralyzed due to fear and worry. When we're in the valleys of life, often all we see are the mountains on both sides that appear insurmountable to us. But, too often we miss the fertile ground found in the valleys. God allows us to pass through the valleys to refresh us for the climb.

> "If you're going **through** hell, keep going."
> *– Winston Churchill*

Our son wore his LiveStrong bracelet for a long time as a reminder that the race isn't over. Perseverance is key in *all* the trials of life, not just cancer. God calls us to both live strong and finish strong.

> *"Not that I have already obtained all this, or have already arrived at my goal, but I press on to take hold*

*of that for which Christ Jesus took hold of me. Brothers and sisters, I do not consider myself yet to have taken hold of it. But one thing I do: **Forgetting what is behind and straining toward what is ahead, I press on toward the goal to win the prize for which God has called me heavenward in Christ Jesus.**"* Philippians 3:12-14

What if I die?

"All the days ordained for me were written in Your book before one of them came to be." Psalm 139:16

Each one of us has a specific number of days allotted to us by God. None of us know if we have been ordained with a short, medium, or long life. The fact is, whether we live 49 or 94 years, it goes by fast!

"What is your life? You are a mist that appears for a little while and then vanishes." James 4:14

"Show me, O LORD, my life's end and the number of my days, let me know how fleeting is my life. You have made my days a mere handbreadth; the span of my years is as nothing before You. Each man's life is but a breath." Psalm 39:4-5

I have heard it said, "We are invincible until the day the Lord takes us home." The only thing that matters is that we live each day well. Psalm 90:12 says,

"Teach us to number our days aright, that we may gain a heart of wisdom."

We've all heard the question, "If you knew you only had a week to live, how would you spend it?" Since we *don't* know how many days we have on this earth, we need to ***live*** like there is no tomorrow, with great abandon and fearlessness, all for the glory of the Lord!

> *"If we live, we live for the Lord; and if we die, we die for the Lord. So, whether we live or die, we belong to the Lord."* Romans 14:7-9

Whether our cancer (or any health issue) ends in physical healing here on earth or complete healing in heaven (for followers of Jesus Christ), we need to finish the race of life victoriously.

> *"For I am already being poured out like a drink offering, and the time has come for my departure. I have fought the good fight, I have finished the race, I have kept the faith. Now there is in store for me the crown of righteousness, which the Lord, the righteous Judge, will award to me on that day—and not only to me, but also to all who have longed for His appearing."* 2 Timothy 4:6-8

The Apostle Paul sums this chapter up perfectly, so I will let Him close with this wise perspective on life:

> *"For we know that if the earthly tent we live in is destroyed, we have a building from God, an eternal house in heaven, not built by human hands. Meanwhile we groan, longing to be clothed instead with our heavenly dwelling, because when we are clothed, we will not be found naked. For while we are in this tent, we groan and are burdened, because we do not wish to be unclothed but to be clothed instead with our heavenly dwelling, so that what is mortal may be swallowed up by life. Now the one who has*

fashioned us for this very purpose is God, who has given us the Spirit as a deposit, guaranteeing what is to come. Therefore we are always confident and know that as long as we are at home in the body we are away from the Lord. For we live by faith, not by sight. We are confident, I say, and would prefer to be away from the body and at home with the Lord. So we make it our goal to please Him, whether we are at home in the body or away from it." 2 Corinthians 5:1-9

~9~

DIAGNOSIS AND CURE FOR THE #1 KILLER

M aybe you bought this book, or someone gave it to you, because you are going through breast cancer, but you don't know Jesus Christ as your Lord and Savior. Maybe you even thought, "That's *a lot* of talk about Jesus, but I'll get through this with my positive thinking and determination. Religion is fine for her, but that's not my thing."

Maybe you simply have never been properly "introduced" to Jesus prior to reading this book. Hopefully, after finishing it, you *do* want to know Him in an intimate way, but you simply don't know how.

Please allow me to share with you the plan and purpose of Jesus coming to earth. He came just for you!

Our life on earth is a terminal condition! There is a 100% chance that we will all die one day. That's a given, but there are only two possibilities relating to where we go once this life is over. The Bible is very clear that we'll spend eternity in either Heaven or Hell. You may think that when this life is over, that's it, there is no more. But, that's not what Jesus Himself tells us. He warned His listeners more about the horrors of hell than He talked about the splendor of heaven.

"For God so loved the world that He gave His one and only Son, that whoever believes in Him shall not perish but have eternal life. For God did not send His Son into the world to condemn the world, but to save the world through Him. Whoever believes in Him is not condemned, but whoever does not believe stands condemned already because he has not believed in the name of God's one and only Son." John 3:16-18

"He is patient with you, not wanting anyone to perish, but everyone to come to repentance." 2 Peter 3:9

Our sin separates us from God. It's like cancer coursing through your body destroying everything in its path, "flying under the radar" for a long time. We often don't detect it until it is pointed out through more careful examination, like a mammogram. It **will** kill us if we do nothing. That's why when we hear the words "You have cancer", our normal response is to kick into high gear and take extreme measures to eradicate it from our bodies. We have an innate desire to live. You certainly wouldn't be satisfied if the doctor performed surgery on you and told you that he removed "most" of the cancer and concluded with, "Let's hope for the best", and sent you home. But that's just what we do in our lives before we put our trust in Jesus as our Savior; we try to clean up our act and hope our good deeds outweigh the bad, hoping that God will somehow grade on a curve and let us into Heaven. That's not the way it works!

"Jesus said to her, 'I am the resurrection and the life. He who believes in Me will live, even though he dies; and whoever lives and believes in Me will never die. Do you believe this?'" John 1:25-26

We can't get rid of cancer on our own. We need all kinds of doctors and specially-formulated medicines and radiologists and machines to check and see if it is all gone. Even if you are using alternative medicine treatments, you are still counting on something else to cure you. That's how it is with our eternal life. We can't play doctor and cure ourselves. We can't be good enough or try harder to earn our way into Heaven. Just one sin keeps us from being able to enter into God's perfect heavenly home. We need "the" cure! It is our only hope for our future...for life. Jesus is called the 'Great Physician'. He is the prescribed way that God has provided for us to be "fully healed" and to have life everlasting with Him. John 14:6 says,

"Jesus answered, 'I am the way, and the truth and the life. No one comes to the Father except through Me.'"

In the case of salvation, there is no alternative cure for our fatal disease of sin.

"The wages of sin is death, but the gift of God is eternal life in Christ Jesus our Lord." Romans 6:23

It's as if the doctor told you, "Your cancer is terminal. You *will* die; it's just a matter of time." At that moment a stranger came in the room and said, "Not so fast. I will take your cancer and die in your place so you can live. But you must fully trust me for this to work." How amazing would *that* be?! Well, that's exactly what Jesus Christ has done for us. He took on *all* of our sin and died willingly on the cross for each of us so we could be made whole and acceptable to God.

"Therefore, if anyone is in Christ, he is a new creation; the old has gone, the new has come!" 2 Corinthians 5:17

The only question is; will you accept this free gift of God's grace?

"Everyone who calls on the name of the Lord will be saved." Romans 10:13

"If we confess our sins, He is faithful and just and will forgive us our sins and purify us from all unrighteousness." 1 John 1:9

Which will you choose: eternal life with God, surrounded by His love and goodness, or eternal separation from Him, miserable and plunged into utter darkness? The choice is yours. God doesn't send anyone to Hell; each person chooses their own eternal destination. Each one of us must decide whether we want God's will for our lives or demand our own will.

"But when the kindness and love of God our Savior appeared, He saved us, not because of righteous things we had done, but because of His mercy. He saved us through the washing of rebirth and renewal by the Holy Spirit, whom He poured out on us generously through Jesus Christ our Savior." Titus 3:4-6

Accepting Jesus Christ as your Lord and Savior is a win-win proposition! He cures you of your fatal disease of sin and He heals your soul. There are many side-effects though: Love, joy, peace, hope, eternal life, becoming a new creation, having a personal relationship with God, losing your fears and replacing them with faith... and the list goes on and on! The promises of God are never-ending. I pray that you will claim your first promise from Jesus today:

"Whoever comes to Me I will never drive away...For My Father's will is that everyone who looks to the

Son and believes in Him shall have eternal life." John 6:38-40

Jesus is inviting you into a life-changing relationship with Him. He says, *"Here I am! I stand at the door and knock. If anyone hears My voice and opens the door, I will come in."* Revelation 3:20

I pray that today will be the day you begin an exhilarating adventure with Jesus and *"take hold of the life that is truly life."* (1 Timothy 6:19)

"The LORD is near to all who call on Him, to all who call on Him in truth. He fulfills the desires of those who fear Him; He hears their cry and saves them." Psalm 145:18-19

Breast Wishes,

Karen

Printed in the USA
CPSIA information can be obtained
at www.ICGtesting.com
LVHW051046010823
753807LV00009B/15